ANGEL
ARE NOT JUST
FOR CHRISTMAS

CAROLEANNE AND MICHAEL JOHNS

ISBN No: 978.1.906542.25.2

Publishers: Barny Books
                 Hough on the Hill
                 Grantham
                 Lincolnshire
                 NG32 2BB

                 Tel: 01400 250246
                 www.barnybooks.biz

Printed by: Spiegl Press Limited
                 42 Guash Way
                 Ryhall Road Industrial Estate
                 Stamford
                 Lincolnshire
                 PE9 1XH

                 Tel: 01780 762550
                 www.spiegl.co.uk

Cover illustrated by Roger McKay

Every effort has been made to describe our experiences that occurred fourteen years ago, however, some experiences have been blurred due to the passage of time but all events are true. The names of the authors and children have been changed in order to respect confidentiality.

2

Acknowledgements

We would like to thank Molly Burkett (Barny Books) for her faith and courage in us and for asking us to write this book.

We send a big thank you to all the members of the Workers Educational Association for their ongoing support, a special thanks to our tutor, Becky Cherriman for her guidance and tuition in the art of Creative Writing. Michael would also like to thank the "Wharfedale Writers" for their ongoing support.

Thanks to our Link Worker and all the team from Family Placement who helped to organise all the excellent training and support. We would also like to thank our own four children for their patience and support during the last twenty years.

And finally, we would like to thank all the many children who put their trust and faith in us and allowed us to share in their lives. It has been a real pleasure.

Michael and Caroleanne
January 2010

Note about the authors.

Michael and Caroleanne became professional Foster Carers in 1996 working with a Family Placement Service which provides a flexible service in order to meet the needs of disabled children and their families.

Both Caroleanne and Michael had extensive experience working with children who were being 'looked after' by the Local Authority. Michael continued in this role until he was able to gain his degree in Play Work, Caroleanne was able to start her own business as a Counsellor and Reiki healer after she obtained her degree.

They both experienced the trials and joys of step family life and, as a result, they became fully trained telephone counsellors giving them the confidence to support birth families of the various foster children.

Caroleanne and Michael felt they had something to offer disturbed and vulnerable children after witnessing other children's experiences of living in Children's Homes. They felt the environment did not suit some children.

Michael had heard about the service offered by Family Placement through his contacts at work. They offer a fee to one person which enables them to give up their full time job.

Michael and Caroleanne first met over twenty years before they formed a relationship. Both worked for a voluntary organisation in the early seventies. Michael had left the Navy and Caroleanne had begun her working life after college. At that time they knew little of each other. However, a year later, when Caroleanne was leaving to get married, Michael invited himself to her hen night! Years later they met again at a local dance and began to form a lasting relationship. They have two children each from previous marriages. This found them dealing with problems of reconstituting a new family.

They both believed that becoming carers would not prevent them from fulfilling their dreams of seeing the world and obtaining first class degrees. They were each able to start their own businesses.

Caroleanne has been interested in life's connection with the angels for some considerable time prior to meeting Michael. However, Michael soon caught up once he had witnessed some of the events described in this book. The couple visit Glastonbury on a regular basis in order to fill up their spiritual tank.

They both believe that, without a 'higher power', they would not have succeeded in their role as foster carers. Hence the birth of this book; the rest, as they say, is history.

WHEN THE CHILDREN ARE ASLEEP

"I've talked about angels to a lot of people now and feel that is what angels want."
An Angel On My Shoulder   Cheung, T (2008)

His temper tantrum had been going on for an hour. The language flowing out of the bedroom would make a sailor blush. It certainly surprised me as he was so young. We could hear the wailing from the kitchen. I had just finished a shift at the Hostel where I worked and was hoping for a peaceful evening. No chance!

Never under estimate a child with a learning disability. I glanced at Caroleanne who looked back at me with concern and worry.

"It's your turn I've been trying to settle him for an hour."

I took a deep breath as I made my way upstairs to the bedroom. It was nine thirty on a bleak Saturday evening and Mark, aged six and three quarters, was refusing to settle. I began to think that something must have happened when he was at home.

Mark had been coming to stay with us for the last three weekends and had never been a problem at bedtime. Caroleanne had been up and down stairs all evening. Now it was my turn. We tended to work in shifts. Sometimes we discovered that children will respond to a 'new' face and Caroleanne and I had learnt to withdraw from a conflict situation in order to enable the other person to try and calm it.

I tried to settle Mark by offering to read him a story. He rejected this idea by throwing his pillow on the floor and started to jump up and down on the bed. He then started to play the 'light switch' game. He was quick to learn how to test our limited boundaries. It had been a very busy day and I was wondering why I found myself in this situation. What had I done to deserve this on a Saturday night? The honeymoon period was definitely over. My patience was running out fast. Mark knew he was well on the way to the 'winner's enclosure' and I was running out of options.

"What shall I try next?" I wondered.

5

There is a foster parent manual of common sense that clearly states that if at first you don't succeed, take a deep breath and try something else but be quick about it. With this tactic firmly tuned into my tired brain, I found myself reluctantly asking Mark if he wanted to follow me downstairs. I decided it was important to have a last word which was not always an easy thing to achieve in Mark's case.

"If you promise to be quiet you can watch TV for thirty minutes, but first you must tidy your bed." Mark gave me one of his charming smiles that could melt an iceberg and he quickly obliged. It wasn't long before he began to calm down. Caroleanne was waiting for him holding a drink of hot chocolate. Within twenty minutes Mark was asleep on the settee.

Conflict often started with our foster children either at bedtime or when having a meal around a table. These settings were an ideal battleground and each child had their own way of gaining attention at crucial moments.

Whilst employed as a Care Officer in children's homes, I had to deal with this kind of situation many times. Those in similar situations knew there was immediate support, especially if a child became too volatile or violent. In a foster home you are on your own and you have no choice but to rely on your experience and training. You have no one to consult until the Social Workers return to their desks. There was an emergency system in place if things got really difficult but we never had to use it.

"HOME SWEET HOME"

In Mark's case, his meals at home had been placed on a saucer and put on the floor by his mother who rarely checked to see if her son ate the food. He had no routine to follow at bedtime so would often sleep on the floor until Mum picked him up and took him to bed. Because of this we dropped all ideas of imposing a set bedtime for a short while to allow Mark the time to adapt to his new environment. The week after the unsettled weekend, we found that

6

Mark's birth father had paid Mum a visit. We guessed this visit hadn't gone well. Dad had a history of domestic violence.

Various behaviour plans were introduced during this time. We were short term foster carers. With patience and perseverance coupled with some excellent support from our Link Worker, we managed to maintain a structure in our home without having to make judgements on what parents did or did not do in their own home. All the children we cared for always wanted to return home no matter what the environment was like.

"SILENCE IS GOLDEN"

It is a good feeling when the house finally falls silent and we reflect on the day. We would feel a sense of achievement and begin to realize the scale of our commitments made to the eleven children who had been coming to us for short breaks and what it meant to them.

We looked after a number of children who had no way of expressing the anger and frustration that was inside them. We spent a lot of time discussing these issues with other professionals and agreed a strategy with them and the child. Sometimes the birth parent would listen to us but often the child went back to a routine which was totally different to our own.

"Some religions believe we all have one or more personal angels allotted to us at birth, to act as spiritual guardians, watching over us and preserving us from harm." Eckersley, G.S. (1996)

CAROLEANNE'S STORY

The threads of experience which ran through my childhood shaped my life in the later years. As a child I was in a constant state of confusion in need of love and support which for most of the time was not there. I was brought up in a busy house and there was a family business to run. My mother was eager to work with my father

7

so she returned to work as soon as I began school. My elder sister had been planned and was born shortly after the end of the Second World War. I arrived three years later and this was not planned, in fact I was a shock as my parents had just wanted the one child. I grew up knowing this.

It always felt like such a long walk to school. The other children were taken by their mothers and I would latch on to them. I remember the feelings of inferiority. In adulthood I realized working in the family business was where my mother found her own self confidence. At that time it was quite unusual for women to go out to work. I was obviously a sensitive child and felt things deeply.

When the time came for me to choose a career, I chose Child Care, Residential work appealed. I felt an affinity with children whose needs were great. I could identify in some ways with many of them. I also felt this was really satisfying work and more selfishly it could mean working away from home. The need to escape the 'family' was by now a very strong need within me. We were required to have placements in various children's homes. I loved the work being busy with the daily routine, the cooking and all things domestic. I also found the behaviour of many of the children so interesting that I was spurred on to study child psychology. I was always aware of the child who hides away, the child who gets ignored as they are so quiet they almost disappear. During my first marriage, I had wanted to foster children. It was a compulsion within me. My first husband would not entertain the idea. I was bringing up our own family at the time so I could understand that maybe it was not the right time to take this on. Second time around and twenty years later I had a clear idea of what I felt my purpose in life was. I met someone who shared the same work background as me and so much more. A great sense of humour is a wonderful thing to share. Throughout all the ups and downs, the stresses and strains, we have never lost this art of laughing together. When we get near to losing it, we take ourselves off for what we call our 'foster carers day out' until our humour returns.

I always wanted to run my own show. I do not like to be told what to do. Fostering children has given me an opportunity to develop my independent spirit. I worked in various institutions in the past but my nature always came into conflict with the style and management. I knew I could do better. I have developed "high standards" and, in my opinion, some of the places I have worked in have failed to meet my own expectations. During my initial training in residential childcare I went on an escorted visit to a children's home for disturbed boys. I was shocked at the stark surroundings which echoed the treatment the boys were receiving. I was upset by the bleak living conditions which lacked any warmth or home comforts. This vision remained with me and helped me create my own approach which is very different to this.

When Michael explained to me that I could chuck in my job as a Care Officer, I leapt at the opportunity. The Family Placement system paid a fee and salary for looking after disabled children. I could plan my own life around the needs of the children and there were many benefits for us as a couple.

This was a wonderful opportunity. Michael and I had always had a creative approach to life. This often involved lateral thinking. We could view our journey into fostering as a total way of life rather than just a means to earn a living. The expenses and allowances we earned were viewed as an added benefit and allowed us and our foster children to lead a good life. This involved weekly outings, wonderful holidays to long haul destinations as the scheme provided us with forty days respite holiday a year and day to day financial security.

I had the opportunity to study for a degree which had always been a wish. I have never regretted my decision to become a foster carer.

MICHAEL'S STORY

I have often been asked why I decided to be a foster carer. The thought never entered my head until I met Caroleanne. Even then I was reluctant to share my newly married life with other people's children. I thought angels were what you sang about at Christmas. These thoughts stayed with me until I began to care for children with disabilities. It is these children who gave me the incentive to feel that I could make a difference to a child's life. I also wanted to prove that a man could love and care for other people's children. Every time I picked up a newspaper there was a story splashed over the pages of a man who had been accused of abuse or viewing child pornography. I don't recall ever seeing a positive story about men. The male species was getting a bad press! When I started fostering I began to witness 'miracles' occurring in my own home.

My early childhood was unsettled so I joined the Royal Navy when I was fifteen. My parents split up some years later and I found myself in a situation where I had to choose between two homes. My Mum had moved to a small flat and had little spare space for me. My Dad was seriously ill and eventually lost his battle against cancer. I was forced into selling the family home which left me feeling homeless.

I became a Care Officer working in children's homes shortly after leaving the Navy in 1972. I was offered full board in return for working a hundred hours plus a week. I began to learn my trade the hard way whilst working for The National Children's Home. The unsocial hours played havoc with my social life but I worked alongside experienced staff who knew their business and I quickly learnt how to look after "the whole child" learning how to cook, sew and iron.

Ten years later I was transferred to a hostel that cared for children with disabilities where I was introduced to the Family Placement scheme which Caroleanne and I eventually joined.

I settled into this environment very quickly after learning how to cope with children who had severe disabilities and were doubly incontinent. I was extremely comfortable working with special needs children and their families and I was immensely relieved at being away from the mainstream Children's Homes.

When I was studying for my degree in Play Work, I became aware of a horrific statistic that states there are over 2 million children living in England and Wales will grow up without meeting a male role model.

I'm glad I changed my mind about becoming a foster parent. The decision never stopped me doing what I wanted to do. In fact, it was just the opposite. The experience has provided me with the opportunity to change my career and start my own business.

THERE'S A BRIGHT GOLDEN HAZE ON THE MEADOW

July 1996 - The Early Years

So here we were with this our first fostering encounter:
We were excited. At long last the time had arrived when we would meet our first child. Mark was aged six going on twenty; he was a mixed race child whose cheek matched a loud gob that had an answer for everything. We loved him to bits. He was our first child on the short term foster scheme. He was to come for one weekend a month. We had to collect him from school on a Friday evening and return him the following Monday.

"Do you sleep in the same bed as him?" Mark's big voice came over loud and clear to the whole audience in the park café. We had taken him there for our first outing. 'Ground swallow me up', was a common thought when we were with this cute and very cheeky little boy. We soon learned that Mark's early years had been short on attention. He had developed his shouting, gobby voice to get heard. My own childhood had been similar in some ways. There were parallels to be made. Mark's reaction to his childhood was to fight. In my own life as a child I had the flight response. I had almost disappeared.

We became approved for the fostering scheme after jumping through lots of hoops. The whole process took about twelve months. It involved our Key worker visiting us on a regular basis. She interviewed us as a couple and then in separate rooms in order to assess motivation. Our Link Worker played an important and supportive role. We had shared our own personal experience, this established a mutual trust which was important to me. We viewed our experience with Family Placement as absolutely positive.

She then interviewed all the friends who had given us references. During the process we attended various courses: 'Child Protection', 'The Children's Act', 'Dealing with Challenging Behaviour' and 'Attachment Theories' to name a few. We began to learn that we would have to form a partnership with the child's birth family.

12

Once our application was completed, it had to go to a Panel whose role is to approve all Foster Carers. It was a nerve racking experience as we waited with fingers crossed for the panel's decision. If it went against us the appeal process would be long and arduous.

The paperwork we received on Mark seemed fairly straightforward. The initial experiences failed to match what we had read. This was quite often the case. Children behave differently in various surroundings and are also different with different people.

He arrived mouthing off and never shut up even for a minute. He demanded attention from the second he got out of bed until he returned to it at the end of the day.

Mark and I were in the car, I had planned an activity packed day with him as Michael was working. He was sitting in the back and his language began to get rude. I was playing his favourite music on the stereo and encouraging him to sing along. But no, he preferred to splutter rude expletives at me, repeating the same things over and over again. I found it impossible to detach my mind from his very loud voice. I had to stop the car. It no longer felt safe to continue driving. I swore under my breathe feeling frustrated at myself that this child could wind me up like this. I talked myself into getting a grip on the situation. We had been on our way to a local farm park to see the animals. I needed to demonstrate responsibility for actions. In spite of the fact that this would be harder on me than him, I turned the car around and we returned home. There would be no farm park and no trip to MacDonald's afterwards.

This was early days with Mark and firm boundaries needed to be established. As we got to know him we realised what a complex character he was. One minute he was all angelic listening to his favourite stories, 'Animals of Farthing Wood'. Within the next half hour he would be supposedly play fighting and would be tough and oblivious of his own physical pain and also capable of throwing really hard punches on to his unwilling victim with whom he was 'playing'.

13

It was a challenge to encourage him to sit at a table to eat a meal. He would be up and down and all over the place. He totally ruled the roost at home. Mum was exhausted.

His behaviour began to concern us so we introduced our first behaviour plan which was centred on a 'Star Book' and 'Star Chart' (see Useful Information page 59) this combination worked well. Mark loved going to McDonald's. A trip was an ultimate reward for consistent good behaviour. He also responded to 'one to one' reading sessions, especially with Michael. Mark's father had disappeared when he was a few months old. So having one to one time with a positive male was a good experience for him. Initially Mark came for one weekend a month however, as Mum became more confident in us and realised her own inability to cope with her family situation, he actually spent weeks at a time with us on a regular basis. . I remember that Mark's ambition in life was to drive a dustbin lorry.

Our second child to come for respite care was Bobby. Initially it was necessary for us to visit the family in their home as it was difficult for them to travel. The family consisted of two disabled children plus two siblings who were non disabled.

I was shocked at the living conditions of this family. The walls had no wallpaper and there was no floor covering on the stairs. It was difficult to sit down as all the chairs were dirty and full of clothes and toys. Their Social Worker explained that they were a very loving family who were on a list to be re-housed. This was a family in real need of help. Mum and Dad appeared very caring of each other. They were obviously living in extreme poverty.

Bobby was extremely thin and had been a 'Failure to Thrive' child, mainly caused by the work load presented to his overworked Mum. He had been underweight throughout his young life. It could be a sign of possible neglect of some kind.

He would spend one weekend a month with us. I made sure I fed him really well with plenty of extras in an effort to build him up. The family were fine to work with. I was interested in looking after

14

Simon's elder sister who was profoundly disabled but Michael had some concerns about administering rectal diazepam. This is an invasive treatment used for severe epilepsy and required specialist training and would normally be administered by a same sex carer or a nurse. This situation would not always be possible in our family.

Bobby was a nice enough lad who would seek extra attention by stealing things from our house. He wanted to give his Mum a present. Nothing of any value was ever taken.

By this time we were feeling settled into the scheme and all was progressing well. On one occasion we had shown an interest in taking on a particular child. The family of the child rejected us. The Social Worker told us it was because we had both been divorced. This seemed odd to us living in times when it is more the norm.

We were asked to take on a toddler for respite care. His family lived in an overcrowded house on a nearby estate. The family had just had a new baby. The parents seemed very young themselves. I observed the mother treating this baby like a doll. It was dressed up in frilly clothes but the baby did not look that clean or comfortable. We did the usual phasing in of the little boy, Alan. On his first evening with us he toddled in front of the television and began to masturbate. We diverted his attention with toys and games. I later visited his special school and worked with the teachers. They were fully aware of the situation, and were being supportive to the family. One evening whilst Alan was with us the telephone rang. It was Alan's mum I reassured her that Alan was fine.

"I've dropped the baby," she said. They never called the baby by its name, just 'baby'.

I asked her if the baby was hurt. She said she didn't know. I suggested that she take the baby to casualty as they lived quite near the hospital. After talking to her for a while she assured me she would do this. I then rang the emergency duty team to report the incident as I was feeling very uneasy. A few weeks later we were out at the fair in the city centre when we saw the parents enjoying the fair without any children with them. They were very young and had special needs themselves. Social Services were fully aware of the

15

situation. There was little else we could do. Our role was to support where we could and the child with us was our concern. In order to do this, we had to let go of any emotional worry and act in a professional manner as this is our survival mechanism when involved in a difficult job. Eventually the children within this family did transfer to long term foster homes which I can only say was the best outcome.

While Michael was working in a short term respite unit, he met two brothers. Michael had met the parents on many occasions and they had expressed their concerns about the unit being too large to meet the needs of both their sons. Phillip and James had been diagnosed with 'Fragile X' which is a condition on the Autistic Spectrum. Michael felt that the boys would fit in well with us. The introductions went ahead. All went well and Phillip and James came to live with us for a weekend a month for over eight years. James the eldest was kind to his brother and seemed easier to communicate with. Phillip the youngest was quite nervous and relied on his brother for his security. We understood that being away from their close family was difficult for them. We always made sure that we had an action packed programme of activities when they came.

The boys never gave any eye contact and little feedback as to whether they were enjoying themselves. James, at 17 years old, was obsessed with 'Star Wars' so we familiarised ourselves with the light and dark characters. After a weekend of talking and acting out the battles, we felt quite exhausted when Monday morning arrived.

On the rare occasions when we met the whole family in a shopping centre, Phillip and James would completely ignore us and not even look at us or even speak. Although we did understand the reason, it still felt tough being ignored.

The information about us would be passed on to the birth parents and, if they agreed, a meeting would be arranged. They would visit us in our home and, over tea and cake, we would find out more about each other. We were always aware of just how important this first meeting was. We began to understand that it was hard to allow another family to look after your child. Quite often members of the birth family would make an excuse to visit us at weekends or while we were engaged in activities.

Prospective parents would be tired out and in need of a break; however, they would remain unable to trust anyone else to care for their child. We would meet and go through the process but often in the end the parent was unable to let go.

If all the families involved were happy then tea time visits with the child would be arranged. There was no set plan for this. It was very much an individual situation. Each child is different and it can take some longer than others to settle. These short visits progressed to an overnight stay and eventually plans were made for a weekend stay. This was monitored closely so that the child was happy and felt safe in their new situation.

'CLIMB EVERY MOUNTAIN'

"There are only two ways to live your life. One is as though nothing is a miracle. The other is as though everything is a miracle." Albert Einstein

We were approached by our Link Worker and asked if we would like to offer emergency and Out of Hours placements. This would mean that children would turn up at short notice. They would arrive with little or no information.

The day dawned with a promise of sunshine. I woke slowly and the daily plans gradually filtered into my mind.

I needed to get up quickly today, not the usual laze with a much needed coffee. Today the social worker was bringing an eight year old girl. She was coming to us at short notice due to some sort of emergency that the social worker had not gone into. I had little information but having had many boys coming to us, I felt excited that at last a girl was coming to stay.

The day unfolded and it became quite warm. I laid out rugs on the grass and added a few activities.

Ruby looked beautiful with her black skin and her hair piled up into a pony tail. The social worker had obviously worked hard dressing her up so she looked her very best. She had to be carried in as she is a wheelchair user. We had steps into the house so access with the chair proved difficult. Ruby was quite agitated on arrival. There had been no time for the usual phasing in or even to meet her beforehand. This must have felt difficult for her. This visit initially lasted for two weeks. She remained with us for ten years.

We placed her on the lawn. The social worker left and I spent the day getting to know her. I had a strong feeling even then that this was going to be life changing. During those initial two weeks, we had many visits from people from Ruby's school who were obviously concerned about her. The school nurse was very attentive. At the time I felt she was interfering, however, it was a tribute to Ruby that the staff in school wanted her to have a good home and were rooting for her in many ways.

Of course we did need some advice on what she liked and disliked although she taught us all those things very quickly. Doing her hair was one of the most difficult things. I did not know anyone with a West Indian ethnicity so had no one to consult. We ended up going to the local market and asking a West Indian lady's advice. She gladly pointed us to a stall that sold specialised hair products. Over the years we had some adventures over her hair. On one occasion I had found a hairdresser who would come to the house. We were thinking of beading and extensions.

The hairdresser did not arrive at the agreed time. It was getting on for eight thirty and still no show. I got Ruby showered and ready for bed. Then the hairdresser arrived. I said that it was too late! In fact she had come a long way on the bus. She said she could do Ruby's hair while she was in bed. So that is what happened. Ruby absolutely loved it.

The whole process took four hours. After it was finished we placed a mirror for her to see. Her eyes lit up. It was obvious how thrilled she was with it.

The information we had received stated that Ruby had been placed with several other foster parents prior to arriving on our door step. She had refused to settle with any of them. It was pass the parcel. Family Placement required a bed for Ruby while they approached other suitable full time carers. There was no room at the Inn. We started to discuss the possibility of transferring to the Long Term Scheme. This scheme offered a fee to enable one of us to give up work. It also offered forty days respite for all carers. We were fortunate to be allocated a wonderful respite carer who had been a carer since the birth of the scheme. Mary was one of the few people who had a ground floor extension so was always busy.

During the fostering training there was a discussion about children who scream a lot. I remember clearly thinking I could not cope with a child who constantly screamed. So how strange and amusing (slightly) that Ruby did scream both through the night and often during the day. This behaviour lasted for two years. We had to learn to interpret her behaviour. I guess Ruby was "training us". My own daughter Victoria helped me so much during those early days. When I was worn out she would help me out by giving Ruby some one to one attention.

Ruby's determination impressed me so much. It was her strong spirit and wonderful sense of fun that amazed me. I soon began to develop a strong bond with her. The change in Ruby's behaviour was gradual as she slowly began to trust us. She soon realised that after going away for her short respite breaks, she would return to us. When we attended her school events we could see from her facial expression how pleased she felt that we were there for her just like any child would be. Ruby had not had this experience in her past. So in many ways it was more important.

On reflection I don't think we gave the situation a great deal of thought or realized what an impact Ruby would make to our married

19

life. I had experience of changing pads of doubly incontinent children at the Hostel where I was employed as a Senior Care Officer. I do recall that I was somewhat apprehensive about having to change someone in my own home if Caroleanne was not available which was not very often. However, you will be amazed at the speed that you get used to when doing this necessary task. It became a matter of taking a deep breath and getting on with it. Ruby would quickly become the child we couldn't have by natural means. Over the years a bond developed which has now turned into a real love the power of which is hard to explain.

We had a discussion with her previous carers who told us that Ruby could be a very wilful child who found it difficult to communicate her needs. She was doubly incontinent and had cerebral palsy caused by lack of oxygen at birth. Ruby was a mixed race child whose father had disappeared. Mum was as involved as she could be. Our role was to establish a rapport with Mum who had been suffering from mental illness and was an alcoholic. There were two or three siblings from different fathers all of whom had been placed in Children's Homes or Foster placements. We spent a lot of time and energy ensuring that members of the family remained in contact with each other. Our philosophy was based on our own childhood experiences and some recent statistics that appeared to demonstrate that children in care often lost contact with their siblings altogether. We always knew the importance of family, no matter how traumatic a child's life is at home. Home is what they yearn for. Our commitment to this family was to make sure that they had weekly contact with Ruby. We got to know Ruby's siblings very well over the years. Often the commitment was tested by Mum especially when she turned up at our house the worse for wear and reeking of drink but she loved her children and would do what she could when she came on her weekly visits.

It was our job to transport Ruby to and from Mum's house which was situated on a nearby Council estate. Mum would try to arrange for one of her other children to visit at the same time.

Ruby needed consistency and a routine. It took two years to get her to settle at bed time. Ruby would test our patience to the absolute limit and, on reflection, we feel that a higher power must have helped us or we wouldn't have survived. Ruby had limited communication skills but we intuitively felt that she understood everything that was said to her. I am certainly grateful for the intervention of Caroleanne's daughter who helped out a lot during the nights when Ruby would not sleep. Victoria had the same hair colour as Mum, so Ruby did transfer her affections on to Victoria because of the resemblance. Eventually Ruby began to develop trust in us and her new environment. She began to sleep through the night. I was grateful for Victoria's help as we were both getting exhausted.

Ruby gradually grew in confidence as time progressed. She was getting too heavy to lift up and down the stairs so funding was agreed to build an extension to our house that was fitted with track hoisting and a wheelchair shower. This adaptation was a great help. It also gave Ruby the opportunity to move around the house freely. She was often the first up in the morning and would crawl through the kitchen and navigate herself towards the TV and video and wait until we put her favourite video on. It was during a Saturday morning when I heard Ruby say a complete sentence: "Can I have some sweets and pop please Michael?"

I nearly fell over the rug as I had never heard her speak. Miracles were happening in our own front room. I got dressed as quickly as I could and went to our local shop to comply with her request. It seemed that the years of love and affection were beginning to reap a reward. Caroleanne explained that Ruby had been trying to speak before when I had been at work.

"IT'S BEEN A HARD DAYS NIGHT"

"Another sign that an angel is close by you is a feeling of emotional well being, a feeling of being well cared for."
Cheung T An Angel on my Shoulder (2008)

Monday March ,1998

It was 6.00a.m. I heard a clomping sound at the bottom of the stairway followed by the words: "Caroleanne, Caroleanne", Ruby was awake and telling me it was time to get up.

I lifted my weary body out of bed, grabbed my dressing gown and ambled downstairs. Meanwhile Ruby had made her way into the lounge by crawling on all fours and I found her kneeling in front of the television. I noticed that she was wet through and needed changing. On this occasion she had at least kept her pad on.

"Come on Ruby it is time to get ready for school." She looked up at me with a vague expression but I knew that she could understand what I had said so I repeated my command. "We will be late if we don't get a move on." I opened the lounge door and breathed a sigh of relief when Ruby began to crawl towards her bedroom.

Fortunately we had track hoisting fitted in Ruby's room when the extension was built. We were also lucky enough to have en suite facilities and after a long wait a shower chair arrived.

Ruby was placed into the track hoisting harness and then lowered into her shower chair. Both Michael and I had recently completed a course on 'Lifting and Handling' which gave us the required skills.

"It's time for a shower, Ruby", Ruby always loved her showers as she liked feeling clean. She would smile and cooperate most of the time. Soon it was time to get dressed for school. I offered her two choices of clothes to wear. "Right, Ruby what would you like to wear today?" I said holding up two sets of clothes. She would either point or smile at her choice. I had learnt that Ruby was great at making her own choices. I would then sit her in her wheelchair in front of the

22

television to watch her favourite Teletubbies video. The next task was to wake Simon and supervise his personal care needs which he was capable of doing for himself.

"Simon we are in a bit of a rush today so let's hurry".

"Hello, Caroleanne" Simon would do his best to get ready, he loved school and could not wait to go each day.

Once Simon was done it was time for cereal and a drink just before the transport arrived to take them to their respective schools.

Once the children had left for school it was time for a much needed cup of coffee and checking my diary for the appointments that week. Once I was clear what I was doing it was time to attack the washing. Looking after disabled children always meant lots of laundry each day which included sheets and towels as both could be doubly incontinent. Cleaning the house and making the beds was the next task. I did employ help from time to time to ease the strain. One of my favourite things to do each day was to prepare and cook the evening meal. It was satisfying to see both Ruby and Simon really enjoying their food

At weekends Michael always arranged for the family to eat out in order to give me a break which was most welcome. This was incorporated with various recreational activities which the children enjoyed. We often went bowling and to the cinema. We also enjoyed walks in the countryside. I have fond memories of Rosie our dog pulling Ruby's wheelchair along the pathways. Our dog was a very big help especially when it was hilly.

Ruby had approximately ten specialists involved in her Care Plan. This day I had an appointment with the paediatrician who had agreed to keep Ruby on his caseload. During the early years of caring, the relationship we built up with this paediatrician was important. He knew both children's medical history and had knowledge of their family history. It also meant that any health issue we were concerned about would be taken seriously and dealt with straight away. Neither child had the ability to say if they were feeling unwell, so it was up to me to notice any tiny indicators. If I missed anything it was usually picked up by the staff in school.

On one occasion the paediatrician and the school nurse arranged an immunisation programme at the local football stadium. This was a great incentive. I took Ruby, Simon, Phillip and James then, after they had their jabs, they could have a tour of the stadium. The boys loved it. Simon was particularly frightened of injections so much so that he would try and run away. I made sure he did not see the needle. I wouldn't tell him until the very last minute, then it would be over in a flash. The nurse was aware and we worked together. So the football stadium idea worked a treat for him.

Monday Evening.

It was Caroleanne's night off. It was my turn to look after the children. They would be returning from school soon. It was time to hunt around for a tin of corned beef. I am an expert in cooking "corn beef hash". The children loved it. Well that was my story anyway. I asked Ruby if she had had a good day at school. She held out her left hand and gave me a quick thumbs up sign. I took this as "Yes, Michael."

"Guess what's for tea, Ruby? It's your favourite." I just had time to change Ruby before Simon arrived home. At the time the children were going to different schools which was a situation we were trying to resolve. Simon soon arrived on his school transport. He was brought to the door by his escort.

"Hello, Michael." Simon looked passive and I could hardly hear what he was saying as he stumbled into the hallway. He could be challenging at times.

"Do you want to help me in the kitchen?"

"OK"

"Its corned beef stew."

"That's great."

I dashed into the kitchen to check on my cordon bleu tea closely followed by Simon.

"Can you set the table, please?" We had been showing him how to set a table for months and, more recently, Simon had been doing a good job.

I sat next to Ruby whilst she began to eat her tea. Without warning she threw her spoon on to the floor and started to make a wailing sound.

"Is it too hot for you?" I asked as I picked up the spoon. Caroleanne and I had interpreted this behaviour as a sign that Ruby wasn't hungry. I thought I had made sure that the food wasn't too hot. The second attempt seemed to be successful and Ruby started to feed herself, encouraged by seeing Simon wolf down his portion. Before I could start my own tea, I saw Ruby's hand holding the rim of her plate. Within a split second she threw the whole thing on to the floor creating a terrible mess. She then started to rock back and forth in her wheelchair. She started to wail and scream. I had no choice but to abandon my tea. "No, Ruby. That's naughty! What's the matter?" I decided to wheel her in to the lounge until she calmed down. If the screaming persisted, I would have no choice but to face her against a wall so that she would have no eye contact. Fortunately on this occasion Ruby calmed down very quickly.

"Good girl, Ruby. Good girl." We had learnt during the last eighteen months of Ruby's stay that if she was upset there is normally a reason for it. She could be tired as she wasn't sleeping through the night. She might be suffering from ear ache or have a bad stomach. I had dismissed the fact that her bad mood was anything to do with my cooking. We had a behaviour plan put in place which had been discussed at our last support meeting. It was mainly a case of trial and error. At the time Ruby could not communicate to us verbally. This dramatically improved as her stay progressed.

The children appeared to enjoy watching the soaps although Simon would spend most of his evening staring into space and not concentrating on the television. I tried to engage him in an activity which involved assembling plastic bits together. His interest in this

25

activity didn't last long so we finished up with all of us having a go at playing with picture dominoes.

At eight thirty it was time to see if Ruby would settle for the night. I wheeled her into her room. With some difficulty I started to utilise the track hoisting. It was like something out of the 'Krypton Factor' I was very nervous about using this hoist as it was different to the ones at work. Ruby did her best to cooperate and smiled away when she was hoisted up to her toilet chair. The whole process took me about half an hour. I breathed a sigh of relief when Ruby was safely tucked in bed.

I was looking forward to putting my feet up. I said goodnight to Simon and went to put the kettle on. I grimaced as I heard a familiar clumping coming from Ruby's bedroom. She had got out of bed. I knew I was in for a long night if I wasn't careful. I was glad to hear the sound of our car parking on the driveway. I was saved. Caroleanne was back. I was sure, Ruby was missing her. It didn't take long for us both to work together and settle her down.

Ruby was up and down three times that evening. Good job I had a day off!

'SCHOOL'S OUT TOMORROW'

'Angels don't worry about you. They believe in you.'
Cheung. T "An Angel on my Shoulder" (2008)

We had to attend another meeting at Ruby's school. We were trying to get her moved to the same school as Simon. We felt Ruby's needs were not being met. Until our earlier intervention she had been placed in a group with other children who have profound disabilities. She used to be left in a corner of the class room to loll about on a pile of rubber cushions. Our observations were that she deserved better. We were also unhappy with some of the teaching staff's attitude towards us. We never had the same feeling from any of the staff at Simon's school.

26

When we began to raise the subject of moving Ruby the head began to dig his heels firmly into his office carpet. The schools pet project was a 'Walking Programme' in which Ruby eventually became a full participant. She had been assessed successfully to use a walking frame. Ruby had learnt that she could gain some independence when moving about the school. We recognised this as a great achievement but felt that Ruby would thrive in another school. Simon's school had reassured us that Ruby could carry on with the programme at their school. Several frustrating meetings later we had reached a stale mate.

The next meeting we were supported by a representative from the 'Parent Partnership Programme' who was set up to help people like us to sift through the internal politics of the education system. Once they were involved things moved more quickly and it wasn't long before Ruby moved. In didn't take her long to settle down. The added bonus was that she was able to join in the Summer Play Scheme held every year at the school.

During this period we discovered how difficult it is to change the wording on a child's "Educational Statement". This document is written for children who have been assessed as special needs. It's normally completed when the child is five and stays with them until they reach eighteen. The statement will usually have a list of 'needs' combined with the resources required to meet those needs. It is almost impossible to have this document changed.

SARA'S STORY

"My uncle took me for a ride in his car. I didn't know where I was going. We had to go up some steps. I was feeling frightened because I didn't know where I was. He took me to a flat. I told him I wanted to go home. He was nice to me and gave me a drink and some biscuits. Then some men came. My uncle said; 'Sara, just do as you are told'. I cried that I wanted to go home. He grabbed me and pulled me over to the balcony. He hung me over the edge. I was frightened. He said I had to do what he said or he would throw me over the edge".

Sara came to us on an emergency placement. Carole was relaxing in the lounge one evening after tea. They were all watching TV when Sara suddenly decided to tell her story. In spite of all our experiences we were shocked to hear the details.

She was eight years old.

At that time there were very few girls coming into the system. I could never understand why that was.

Sara would stay with us for a week while all the paper work was completed.

Her eight years had been packed with moments of tragedy. When she began to talk about what had happened I felt ashamed of the human race; especially the male half. Her short life read like a Hammer horror film. In order to make her comply with a gang of paedophiles, they would hang her upside down from the balcony of their flat. It was unclear how she had finished up in this horrific situation but I think members of her family were responsible for the initial introductions and then deserted her.

Sara had an appealing nature in spite of her history and she fitted into our family instantly. However, she hid a dark side to her personality which started to unfold during one of our outings. Sara was very emotionally disturbed so there was no chance of her staying with us longer. I was very sad to see her leave us and I hoped I'd had enough time to demonstrate that all men are not 'bad men' who want to hurt her.

I guess I had strong emotional feelings about caring for Sara. This may well relate to the time I split up from my first marriage when my eldest daughter was eight years old. The marriage had disintegrated a year before I packed my bags and left. I tried everything in order to stay with my two children but it wasn't to be. I was heart broken when Sara left.

DAVID'S STORY

We will always remember our next emergency.

"Would you like to complete an assessment on a child who is causing problems in his family and at his school? A decision needs to be made on which of the fostering schemes he finishes up with."

Our Key Worker had just completed her six weekly visits and casually mentioned the idea. "His name is David and he is twelve years old. I would think he could stay with you for six months. He would then move on to a permanent placement." We readily agreed. We didn't know what we had let ourselves in for.

David's Mum had threatened to throw him out. He had been suspended from school. The situation did not look good. David was emotionally close to his Mum and the long term plan would be for the family to be reunited.

David was one of those children who always had to be right. Black was white. Red was yellow. He was a great braggart who was good at everything. He told Caroleanne he was brilliant at skateboarding. He arrived on our doorstep carrying one that looked brand new. He was a World Champion!

I remember like it was yesterday. We went to our local park where there was a skateboarding area with ramps and all sorts of apparatus to jump from. There were quite a few boys there already. They were showing off their skills. I encouraged David to show me all the things he told me he could perform. He began making excuses. Then his voice started to sound shaky. I twigged how this was going to turn out but felt I needed to pursue it for a while as he had bragged and lied. I asked him to get on the board. I even attempted to get on it myself. This was much harder than it looked and I said as much. By this time he had a crestfallen look on his face and I felt the poor lad had had enough humiliation for one day so told him it was time to go home.

29

We soon realized that David needed structure and discipline and quickly. He also knew which of your buttons to press and, therefore, there were many early confrontations when he tested us out. He would never admit he was in the wrong. When I was in a confrontation with David I had to remember some basic principals learnt when I was a Care Officer. Always keep your hands in your pockets and be prepared to walk away and leave the problem for someone else. Playing the game of 'Good Cop, Bad Cop' would only last for so long. It soon became obvious that we needed to introduce a different strategy. Our earlier experiences with Mark came in very handy. So it wasn't long before we introduced another Behaviour Plan which, thankfully, worked very well.

I had to spend a lot of time at David's school as he was always in some kind of trouble. It was at the time when the 'Inclusion Agenda' was being introduced. This is where some children who would have stayed in a Special School were introduced into main stream education. It became a social policy mantra that some people had not thought this through. A child doesn't necessarily get accepted by his peers and can soon become lonely and ostracised in their new environment. In my opinion, David was one of the 'victims' of the new way of thinking. To be fair the school had scant resources to help square pegs fit into round holes. David was a large square peg (ref: Marsden, R. "The Family Business" B.A.A.F. (2008). He would constantly argue with the teaching staff which was in charge of a class of thirty. In a Special School it would be around twelve. David spent a lot of time in the cooler where he would at least get 'one to one' attention. It was during one of these periods that he was befriended by one of the Assistant Teachers who began to see the 'nice lad' within the struggling and shouting persona presented to other members of staff. Thankfully, Paul lived in the local area so he was ready and able to become a volunteer who would then take David out. This became a godsend and we were extremely grateful for his help.

I had a happy and relaxed childhood until I started to attend Secondary School. It was some kind of a 'culture clash' trying to survive with forty other children in your class. The teachers I remember were mostly strict disciplinarians who did not suffer fools gladly. Sometimes the atmosphere could be very intimidating. But I managed to make some good friends once I bought my first bike. It was due to this background that I had some empathy for the situation that David was in. Although I was never comfortable going into a school, I had to keep reminding myself that I had had as much professional training as the teachers I was dealing with.

David stayed for six months while we completed a full assessment. It was decided that he would be best placed with another carer where he would receive a lot of love and affection. We had learned that David was able to attach himself to another family even though he would have liked to return to live with his Mum. We felt we had given him a helping hand in this direction and David had learnt he could love more than one person.

SCOT'S STORY

Let's meet Scot.

He was a walking, talking human volcano that came to spend the summer holidays with us as his Long Term Family Placement was breaking down.

We had a spare bed for a short time. Scot had been sharing a bedroom with our old friend, David. The two lads were totally incompatible and arguments would often lead to fights which weren't an acceptable situation in a family environment. The summer holidays were six weeks long!

Scot was a fourteen year old, street wise lad who had been around the block a few times. We expected that he would cause us problems but this never happened. One reason for this was definitely the presence of Ruby. Scot and Ruby got on like a house on fire. Scot always offered to push her wheelchair and help manoeuvre it in and out of the mini bus.

Scot informed us that he had a birth sister who had a disability so he was more aware of the difficulties than most people we knew.

Scot had a kind and engaging personality which came out when he was feeling comfortable. He told us about his life in the 'car trade' and disturbing stories about his eldest brother who was in prison for causing grievous bodily harm. He told us that he didn't want to finish up in the same place as his sibling. Scot offered to help if we ever lost our car keys. I think it was his way of giving something back.

Although we felt we were sitting on a volcano, Scot agreed to keep to all our boundaries which were pretty relaxed by then anyway. We had planned a full programme of activities for Ruby and Simon so Scot was used as some extra help which was a role he seemed to enjoy during the short time he was with us. Ruby was always glad to see him. She would say: "Scot, Scot coming."

Scot enjoyed being given responsibility and trust within our home and he responded to this.

He left as quickly as he arrived and we were not sure exactly what happened to him in the long term. Once she had had a long break, his foster mother agreed to give him another go. We hoped he would take some memories of our family life with him.

Because the children and particularly Ruby have special needs, the internal impulse is to protect. So relationships concerning the child and the wider world can take on intensity, particularly with some schools. Trust on both sides needs to be built. In some cases we never managed to achieve this. Over the years this relationship has caused me a lot of stress. There is only communication via a home/school book. Comments can be placed which are so easily misconstrued.

There was one particular time where the comments coming back to us were unsupportive and quite bitchy. This situation had carried on for quite a few weeks. I had spent time at this school in the classroom with Ruby. I had witnessed the staff talking about other parents in an unprofessional negative manner. This attitude was being conveyed to us through this home/school book. One reason was that we witnessed Ruby's heightened awareness of some things which did sound quite remarkable but they were true. At one point it became so bad I rang the headmaster. I was so angry I was crying. He listened to me and eventually, after a meeting, this situation was sorted out.

One reason for this animosity was when we attended another of Ruby's meetings to discuss her progress. Michael and I were telling how Ruby recognised familiar roads and was able to know where she was going on the regular trips we took. This is even though we are many miles away from home. On one occasion we were fifteen miles away from home and we regularly visited a ball pool in a pub. Ruby loved it. When we were about a mile away she began to say, "Ball pool, Ball pool."

At other times when we were taking Simon to his step-mum's she would say "Mummy". The teacher laughed at us refusing to believe what we were saying. We are intelligent people but, as foster carers we were often treated as 'unprofessional'. Ruby used to come out with complex sentences (for her). The only trouble was she only said them once. Working or trying to work with this attitude became more and more difficult. Eventually we felt that Ruby would move on in her development in a different school. We felt that expectations of her abilities would be higher in a different environment. The present school had very low expectations. This was the root of the problems I was experiencing with the school. Within the whole spectrum of disability there is a scale of ability and often it is the carers who read the often tiny signs that indicate a child requires more stimulation at school. We felt that was so in this case. We had to battle for a year to move her. The headmaster dug in his heels. Our own social worker was always very supportive of us. We also gained support from another organisation which was set up to help parents of disabled children. It would seem that parents do have to battle for many things/items they need. It could be a ground floor extension or transport to enable wheelchair access. All of this was provided for us and recognised fully as a standard need. However for natural parents it is a different story. The statistics for parents break up is high due to the strain this puts on the whole family unit. So there are many lone mothers who do the protecting and battling alone. Within the family of a disabled child, the other children can often suffer because there are little energy reserves left. After days, weeks and years of total care, this can take its toll. This is why I felt such a pull to do the respite caring as it supports the other children in the family. They can get a chance of some valuable attention from their family.

'COME FLY WITH ME'

"And sometimes they appear in the guise of other people or animals, consciously or unconsciously guided by those from a higher dimension" Cheung. T. (2008) An Angel on My Shoulder

We were determined that our foster children would have the same experiences as other children so we went on holidays abroad. On this occasion we had decided to fly to the South of France and take our chances with an airline. So fasten your seat belts!

"Will all passengers travelling to Leeds Bradford International Airport on flight NCF 469 please go to Gate 3 and prepare for boarding. Have your passports and boarding cards ready."

The message boomed across the concourse in both English and French. The only problem was that we did not know how we were going to reach our departure gate.

We were retuning from a wonderful holiday at one of the many 'Euro Camps.' Camping in France isn't a cheap option by any means. However, everything is provided.

So there we were trying to fly home from Nice Airport, or so we thought. We were at the tail end of all the other passengers by the time we heard the first announcement. Michael was pushing Ruby in her wheelchair and I was struggling with the hand luggage and supporting Simon who also needed help with his mobility. We arrived at the top of an escalator with Gate 3 obviously at the bottom. We both began to get worried when we saw the last of the other passengers rapidly disappearing through it. The only lift we could find was out of order and we couldn't be sure how long it would have

*taken us to find the alternative route. Time was running out, I
decided to try and get some help so I started to scream. We could
clearly see our plane starting its engines through a large window
and a member of staff checking in the other passengers. My screams
of panic appeared to be ignored. I began to feel everyone was deaf,
very deaf, because we couldn't have made any more noise even if we
had a big drum.*

The second call for passengers to board the plane geared me into
taking some action. I told Caroleanne that I would return to the lift
and double check to see if it had been repaired. I started to bang on
the door. I looked up and saw a notice. Even with my limited French
I could make out directions for Gate 5 which was the alternative
route for people who required assistance. Only problem was I hadn't
a clue how long it would take us all to get there. I returned to
Caroleanne and the children and we both started to bang on the pane
of glass signalling that we needed help. Panic was beginning to take
over my brain cells. How were we going to reach this plane?

I decided to ask a well dressed man for directions to Gate 5. He
looked me up and down as if he was a Sergeant Major giving an
inspection. He hunched his shoulders and with an explosion of
French words turned around and hastily made for a door further
along the corridor. It seemed to me that he wasn't a fan of anything
English. I dropped my shoulders and returned to the top of the
escalator.

*The final call came over the loud speaker system. I was frantic.
"Look, Caroleanne," I heard Michael say, "We'll have to do
something or we'll miss the flight. I'll carry, Ruby on my shoulder
and, with a bit of luck, there'll be a chair down by the gate's
entrance on which she can sit while I find one of the airline staff.
Surely they will help us! I'll come back when I find somebody." I was
so worried that I couldn't speak. So I just nodded in agreement.*

*Ruby was ten at the time. Because of her cerebral palsy and
learning disabilities she has not been able to walk since birth.*

35

However, this was no time to reflect on the problems of lifting and handling. Before I could blink, Michael picked her up, put her across his shoulders and started to go down the escalator. I had no idea what would happen when he reached the bottom. I blinked a tear from my eyes as I saw Ruby's cheerful face beaming and giggling, thinking this was a great game. Ruby knew no fear, as we had found out when we took her on fairground rides.

I watched nervously at the top of the escalator gripping the handles of the wheelchair and saying some reassuring words to Simon who was clinging anxiously to my arm. He is petrified of stairs and is extremely nervous about going down escalators. Before Michael had reached the half way point I heard a voice speaking to me in fluent French. Standing by the wheelchair I was startled to see a tall, elegant man who seemed to be offering his help. I was so surprised, I could hardly speak. All I could do was point to the wheelchair and luggage. The stranger loaded our entire luggage on to the wheelchair and with superhuman effort began his descent down the escalator. I coaxed Simon towards the top step of the escalator. He had been unusually quiet, so I breathed a sigh of relief when he followed me. By the time I joined Michael, Ruby was sitting comfortably in her wheelchair still giggling and smiling. The stranger brushed away our thanks and disappeared through another departure gate. I could not resist giving Michael and Ruby a big hug and kiss. I have never been so glad to see the outline of a plane that was now clearly visible in front of us.

Now we were faced with our next adventure- getting on board the plane. After checking in we were soon ushered into a buggy that had a large platform in the middle where Ruby could sit in her chair. It had four seats which rocked around when the buggy started to move. In a few minutes we reached the underbelly of our plane. We were then greeted by the arrival of a giant machine that I had just seen lifting the luggage into the hold. This device doubled up so that it could be used to help disabled people reach the front door of a plane. A ramp folds down from the front of the machine like a giant tongue. We were beckoned on board by a man dressed in oily overalls. He seized the wheelchair and began to strap it to the floor using two metal clamps. Caroleanne supported Simon whist I found a rail to hold. I am afraid of heights so wasn't looking forward to the experience.

The man in overalls spoke to us in broken English as he instructed us all to hold tight on to the rails at the back of the ramp. The space reeked of diesel and its smell was enough to make me feel ill. One would think that after landing a man on the Moon someone would have invented a better way of transferring disabled people on to a plane.

I held my breath when I heard the squeaking sound of the hydraulic system that clicked into action as we started to rise up towards the entrance of the plane. The lift juggled to a stop and the tongue poked flat out towards the door. At this point Ruby was transferred to a smaller wheelchair that was thin enough to fit the plane's aisle. Two burly men carried her inside towards our reserved places at the front of the plane. Ruby's wheelchair was then removed and stored in the hold. I prayed it would survive the journey as some baggage handlers had little respect for wheelchairs. On one holiday in the Canary Islands, we had to hire another wheelchair because the wheelchair had been damaged when it was loaded into the hold.

It was our job to transfer Ruby to her seat by the window. No airline staff will help you. They are not insured, apparently. However, I was glad to finally be on the plane and in a couple of hours we would be landing and getting ready for the task of getting off the plane, which is more or less the same way we got on but in reverse. I hoped and prayed that Ruby's wheelchair would survive the journey!

'WE'RE ALL GOING ON A SUMMER HOLIDAY'

"There is much evidence of their presence not just within individuals but with larger groups."
An Angel at My Shoulder. True Stories of Angelic Experiences.
(Eckersley, G.S. 1996)

You can't plan for everything when going on a holiday abroad - as our experience at Nice airport clearly showed. To be fair the 'Check In' staff had offered the services of an adapted buggy that would pick us up in the departure lounge. But Caroleanne fancied going around the shops. We would miss all the shops if we accepted this offer.

On a holiday to the Canary Islands we were taken down a dimly lit corridor to wait for our flight in a small, windowless room. The family was a long way from the refreshment hall and accessible toilets. We had to wait for two hours and Ruby became very restless as there was nothing for her to see or do. Then I had my first contact with the dreaded mechanical lift and van which is used to transport rubbish. The airports use this method to transfer disabled people on to a plane. Caroleanne and I didn't want another holiday to end like that.

The children had had a fantastic time in the South of France. I had hired an open top car and we travelled to Cannes and Monaco where we witnessed the 'World Firework Competition' from a vantage point that looked over the harbour. Simon was thrilled to see all the colours and movement in the sky he kept saying, "Wow". All of us were excited about going into the famous Casino and pretending to be James Bond. It was good fun watching other people lose their money.

Simon and I became Stirling Moss when we drove around some of the actual race track as we tried to find our way back to the camp site. We are always getting lost especially in foreign countries. The roads can appear confusing and I find it easy to lose my sense of direction. So things can get quite fraught.

38

We met some wonderful people while on holiday on French camp sites. One memory that sticks in both our minds involved meeting a couple who were teachers. They had three children. Their youngest child was called Brad. He was aged four at the time. He had a terminal illness so his parents were fully employed raising money to help him. We used to get together with them in the evening and share food. It was a great part of our day. Michael and I regret the fact that we lost touch with this family as we found we had a great deal in common. We were invited to visit them on our return to England but only managed to make one trip. They lived near Stratford-on-Avon so we had the opportunity to have a weekend break in beautiful countryside. We discovered the home base of the author of the 'Tellytubbies' which was Ruby's favourite TV characters at the time.

It was Ruby who first met Brad whilst she was befriending a family of ducks which waddled over to greet her every morning. Ruby would have no problem getting out of bed and crawling towards the front door of the tent. She was joined by Simon and they both began to play together before breakfast.

Ruby started to grow in confidence during this holiday and had no problem in striking up a friendship with Brad. This led to an introduction to the rest of the family who were staying in a tent opposite ours. We had a good time having parties in each others tents.

KID'S CLUB

I loved the 'Kid's Clubs' on French camp sites. One of the main reasons is that we had no problems registering Ruby or Simon. Michael took them to the club house on our second day thinking he would have some difficulties in leaving the children. They were accepted straight away and the added bonus was that one of us did not have to stay with them. It was good for their independence not to be with us every minute of the day. This was a totally different experience to any arrangement we had with similar clubs in the UK.

The club was open for two hours, morning and afternoons. The main activities were based on the site so the children were never far away. We could be contacted very quickly if needed. We never were!

Caroleanne and I had just taken the children to the 'Kid's Club' on the morning of our third day. Suddenly we heard the sound of children's laughter and the crash of cymbals and tambourines. We rushed to the door of our tent and our faces lit up as we saw Ruby travelling at speed across the grass being pushed by several children all dressed up as Pirates. Ruby and Simon had had their faces painted and both were sporting a homemade hat. We sat down to drink our tea as we watched this happy crowd of shipmates disappear around the back of the camp site.

Ruby was able to cultivate her friendship with Brad whilst at the club. The children had a wonderful experience long before the 'Inclusion Agenda' was introduced.

'BEACHES'

When looking at holiday brochures my heart skips a beat every time I see a picture of a wonderfully looking wind swept beach with white sand surrounded by a clear blue sky. It doesn't take me long to relax in my chair at home and imagine lying on a sun bed drinking a large cold beer and listening to the loud crashing of the waves as the tide slowly edges in. This wonderful image is soon disrupted by the reality that is imposed on a person who tries to access a beach pushing a wheelchair. My 'World Record' for reaching a beach was about fifty yards in old money. I found myself having to negotiate a large, steep ramp that led to a beach in Majorca. I was pretty exhausted when we finally admitted defeat and had to call a halt. It was a very hot day. We were miles away from the sea. However, this didn't stop Ruby trying to crawl towards the water's edge when we lifted her out of the wheelchair. She has an independent soul and wasn't going to be put off by the distance.

Ruby and Simon both loved playing in the sand which used to get everywhere. The 'Beach Bar' was some distance away. After a couple of hours we decided that we had no choice but to return to the apartments as there were no facilities to change Ruby who was having great fun flopping into beach puddles. Simon would spend hours digging in the sand. He wasn't a lover of water at that time.

We did discover a fully accessible toilet near another beach on the other side of the island so we went there every day that we could in the hired car.

One of the best beaches we found was at Western-Super-Mare, Somerset. The beach is a short drive from the holiday camp. This was a memorable holiday as it was the first one we went on in our newly acquired Jaguar car which we had bought from a private seller. Caroleanne and I had always wanted to own one, so we were over the moon at owning a ten year old Jag we could show off. Simon and I became members of the 'Jaguar Enthusiast Club' and we joined the members on local rallies on runs out to places of interest. On occasion Ruby would join us. She loved that. The members of this club were always friendly and empathic to all our children!

It is possible to drive and park on the sand at Weston-Super-Mare. The beach can then be enjoyed without trailing the wheelchair and buckets and spades. It was also possible to take care of Ruby's personal care needs in the back seat of the car.

One day we parked the car on the beach and enjoyed a few hours of relaxation. When we attempted to leave we discovered we were well and truly stuck. The dry sand had become too soft so the tyres had sunk. The situation was difficult because we owned an automatic car and it wasn't a four wheel drive. So the harder I tried to go anywhere, the worse it became with the rear wheels kicking up sand but refusing to move forwards. We were unsure what to do as there were no other cars nearby. Simon and Ruby were getting hot and bothered by this time. An hour passed before I managed to find a beach attendant who contacted his workmates. They turned up in a tractor and quickly attached a rope to a hook on the front of our 'pride and joy' and started to drag us out. It was a rather ignominious exit for our newly acquired status symbol. Simon thought this was great fun. In fact that was all he spoke about when he talked about this holiday.

HOLIDAY CAMPS

When Ruby became too heavy to carry on to planes, it became time to explore England. We were able to rent a caravan which had been adapted. It had a ramp that led to the front door and it also had a wheel in shower. This was brilliant considering that the charity rented at half price. We enjoyed many holidays in their caravans in many different places. One of the places selected was Burnham on Sea, down the M5 and turn left. Caroleanne and I were able to get permission from the school to travel down in early July so we were able to miss all the traffic. In those days you were allowed two weeks a year.

One particular year we had driven a long way and were looking forward to getting into the caravan, unpacking and just getting on with our holiday. Ruby needed changing after the long journey, but, on arrival the keys were not in the place that had been previously arranged. We decided to have a look at the caravan anyway and sort out the keys when we could get in touch with the charity. To our surprise when we got to the caravan there was a couple from the charity who were waiting for us to arrive. They put the kettle on and produced home made cake. Michael thought how nice this was and I suppose in one way it was very kind. However another part of me felt quite annoyed. All I wanted to do was sort Ruby out and unpack not sit and drink tea with strangers. I felt invaded and patronised. It takes so much effort packing up for all of us, shutting the house up and then a long drive so I would think that most people would just want to get on with their holiday when they finally arrive. The charity was very proud of this new caravan they had just bought. They also probably wanted to check out the people who were staying there. That was the last time we rented a caravan from them though.

One year we took Ruby, Simon plus Simon's sister on holiday to the caravan. The weather was beautiful and we were sunbathing by the pool. Simon joined his older sister for a dip in the pool. I was on my way back from buying an ice cream when I saw a woman grab hold of Simon and holding him quite tightly. She must have thought that he was in some kind of trouble. I asked her who she was.

She stated, "Oh, its fine. I work with the handicapped."

I told her that if this is true then she ought to know better. Our foster children were vulnerable and will attach themselves to strangers very quickly. The person looked upset. I am sure she meant well but I felt her actions were inappropriate. I glanced over at Michael and glared at him, I think he got the message. He had woken up from a snooze. He shrugged his shoulders and stated that Charlotte had offered to look after her brother.

Ruby and Simon loved the entertainments which were based on the site. I took them over quite early in the evening while Caroleanne had a rest. She was not that keen on discos and preferred a good book.

I had to arrange for two members of staff to give me a hand to carry Ruby up to the concert room as the lift was always out of order. We were informed that some children had broken the lift.

We had some lovely evenings together as the children enjoyed relating with all the characters that entertained the children at the Junior Disco. The friendly atmosphere helped Simon and Ruby feel happy and included.

CORNWALL

Cornwall was our next idea for Simon and Ruby's annual holiday. The adapted cottage had been booked. It was situated near the Lizard.

After a few days, the weather was fine and it felt time for a walk along the cliffs. We found a short stretch which we could manage quite easily with the wheelchair. We bought some famous Cornish pasties from 'The Lizard Pasty Shop'. They were just out of the oven and smelt fresh.

We reached our destination which was as far as we could get with the wheelchair. It was very beautiful with the turquoise foaming sea pounding against the rocks. Ruby's face was beaming. She loved the breeze on her face. Simon was enjoying the experience and managing to walk on the uneven ground with some assistance.

Michael seemed very keen to stop and have the picnic. I was thinking it was a bit early to eat. I soon learned the ulterior motive (I should know by now.) Michael just happened to have his radio with him. I had a moan at him. It was so lovely and he insisted on having his radio on. I felt he was spoiling the moment. So off I went in a furious huff. I walked a little way on and nearer the cliff edge to feel the wind which was so bracing and refreshing. The peace was just great.

On my return as I approached Michael who had stayed with the children. I eyed a group of men all gathering around. I thought something must be wrong so I hurried. As I got nearer I heard the sound of the radio commentary. Other walkers had stopped and were all listening to the cricket. Apparently it wasn't just any old cricket match. It was the Ashes and it was a matter of life and death to keep up with the score. So Michael explained as we managed to break free from the crowd of cricket lovers who had found their way to this Cornish cliff. This could only happen to my husband. In the middle of nowhere and he can manage to attract a crowd. I laughed until the tears ran down my face.

It was holiday time again: 'Majorca here we come.' The flight had reached the destination on time and all had gone well. We managed to transfer to our accommodation. By this time we had been travelling for hours. Ruby was doubly incontinent and she really needed to be changed and freshened up after the long journey. When we arrived at the apartments we were told that we could not check in for another two hours. We made a fuss but this got us nowhere. I eventually managed to find a disabled toilet quite a walk away. It was a struggle to sort things but I did manage. The holiday reps were all young and obviously lacked empathy or any understanding of our plight. This situation started our relationship with the holiday reps on the wrong footing.

It was five o'clock in the afternoon, we had just come back from the pool and were getting changed for the evening. A loud knock sounded at the door. I went to answer it. One of the reps stood and then pushed herself into our apartment and began accusing our children of using laser pens in a violent way to other guests. The young rep was certainly in Sergeant Major mode. I was trying to explain to her that our children were not able to use such a device but she was not listening. It took me a few minutes to take in what she was accusing Simon and Ruby of doing. I then walked her over to Simon and Ruby to show her that she was talking to the wrong family. She made no apology for her mistake. After she left we shared a good laugh.

As a treat we had decided to hire an open top car in the belief that both Ruby and Simon would enjoy the experience. Simon loves all things mechanical, especially cars. He engaged with great delight as we drove off. After a few minutes I glanced at Simon through the car mirror. He had his eyes screwed up tightly shut with a sad expression on his face. He did not look as if he was enjoying himself. I checked this out with him and he raved about how great the car was. Simon rarely demonstrates any emotion. His facial expressions often remain set or even in a grimace. We quickly learned that this is no indication of how he is feeling. It is just part of his disability. He has also learned to say the things he thinks you want him to say. It is very difficult to discover just what the reality is for him. Simon's true feelings are expressed through his behaviour. This is because he is incapable of expressing himself in any other way. I did find this quite hard as, more often than not, nothing comes back. Occasionally when we are least expecting it, he will say how he has really enjoyed some outing or activity. That is the icing on the cake.

BEER AND BITTERN

So back to Majorca

Later on in the holiday I had read about a nearby bird reserve where Cattle Egrets were nesting. I thought that Simon would enjoy a walk in the countryside and it wasn't too hot for him on that particular day. We managed to persuade Michael that a trip to a bird reserve wouldn't kill him. Like many blokes, Michael quite enjoys a pint. I was feeling quite pleased with myself that I had found an evening activity away from the many bars and flashing lights.

We reached the reserve and it was decided to take Simon as there were no accessible paths to take a wheelchair. We strolled off with binoculars in hand. Ruby was quite happy sitting with Michael in the parking area, enjoying the fresh evening air, and the plan was to return within the hour.

Simon and I did see the Cattle Egrets nesting in small trees. I also spotted a Bittern which thrilled me, although I don't think Simon was too impressed.

On returning to the car park I could not quite believe what I was seeing. On a bird reserve in the middle of nowhere Michael Johns' had discovered a BEER MACHINE serving ice cold beer. He was sat there knocking it back laughing his head off. After I got over the shock I began to see the funny side of the situation. So did the children.

'IF YOU WANT TO KNOW WHO WE ARE'

"While we are sleeping, angels have conversations with our souls."
Cheung, T. 'An Angel on My Shoulder' (2008)

We had settled into our role as Long Term foster carers for Ruby and Simon.

Once a year on a beautiful summer's day there is an event called 'Opera in the Park'. It is always a wonderful experience as far as we are concerned.

We would pack a picnic with fresh juice for Ruby and Simon and some wine for us. The afternoon is spent getting all the chairs out of the heavily packed storage cupboard. Ruby gets excited and is all giggly and smiling. We drive to the vast park and, along with thousands of others, find a parking spot and plant our picnic box, chairs, and sunhats on to our chosen piece of grass. It is quite a feat. At last we find a nice spot near enough to see but not too near the speakers. We settle the rug and ourselves in our chairs and survey the scene. Ruby loves looking around at all the people. Most are in a really good mood so when she waves at certain faces they usually respond and return the gesture which she absolutely loves. Simon takes life quite differently. He will sit and a smile will hardly ever cross his worried face. Yet later we will hear him telling what a great time he has had. As dusk arrives the music begins, 'The Pearl Fishers' echoes around the park. It is a wonderful opportunity to chill out and look at the sky. It is truly magical. This is yet another example of angels at work. We have never been rained on at this concert yet the one year we were unable to go, it was a total wash out.

One year we were there as usual with thousands of other people. Leaving after the evening is not easy with all the picnic gear pushing a wheelchair and keeping hold of Simon. Without warning we lost Simon in the crowd. We were looking for him in the darkness. We had a word with the security guards and they joined in the search. I decided that I would go to the minibus with Ruby and look round the parked cars. When I reached the minibus Simon was there. It surprised us that he had taken notice of where we had parked and had been able to find his way back..

I then had to go back and let Michael and the security staff know. This incident made us realise that in some ways Simon was more capable than we were aware. This brings up issues of over protection which can limit ability. Whereas when we raise our expectation of ability the individual will use what they are capable of. This was a great learning for us.

SIMON'S STORY

Simon visited us regularly before moving in, coming for tea time visits. On one occasion we went out for fish and chips. Simon responded to the one to one attention he received.

Throughout Simon's early life he was brought up mainly by his stepmother who is a formidable character and is very proud of her family. It is difficult for some members of a child's family to let go. In this case the court decided that Simon had to live in alternative accommodation, so a full 'Care Order' was put in place until Simon reached eighteen. Naturally stepmum wasn't happy about this decision. She has no time for anyone connected with Social Services, which in her mind also included us.

Simon has a younger sister who was also being 'accommodated' in a foster home. We made arrangements for the brother and sister to see each other on regular contact visits. Over the years Simon's sister formed a loving relationship with Ruby. It was great to see them both together.

Simon was very unwell in his early years. When he was a baby he nearly died. Simon has Cerebral Palsy and was diagnosed with Hydrocephalus this means he had to have a shunt fitted inside his brain and a tube is placed in the body in order to drain any fluid away. This disability has caused Simon some considerable problems during his twenty two years.

It is certainly a bonding experience when you find yourself in hospital with a child in the middle of the night. Simon had been complaining of a headache all day. Later he had been sick and turned a weird colour of green. So there we were waiting for him to have a "CAT" scan. Simon is a nervous child so needs lots of reassurance when going through these ordeals. After quite a long wait the Doctors informed me he would need a revision on the shunt fitted inside his head. This device drains the excess fluid away into his stomach. It meant he had a tube drilled into his skull. It was not a pretty sight. Fortunately the hospital has one of the top specialists

48

and the operation was a success. With the help of a wonderful team of nurses and doctors Simon was able to make a full recovery and a week later he was allowed to return home.

.
Years before, whilst I was undertaking residential child care training, we were taken to a ward of children with huge heads. They did not live long lives and were contained in cots with cushions to rest their huge heads on.

How wonderful that the treatment has progressed to such a degree. For most of the time Simon is able to live a full and interesting life in spite of his Hydrocephalus.

When Simon had his 'shunt revision', Caroleanne spent most of her week camped by Simon's bedside. In spite of our concerns it was our job to organise a rota system so that members of the family could visit. I was working full time and we still had to ensure that Ruby received some attention.

On occasion Simon would be physically sick. He would never ever come and tell anyone. We would be left to discover it. Of course the smell came first. You had to hunt it out. A great job cleaning all that up, yuk! This has happened regularly over the years and he still never tells us and never reaches the toilet. We have tried every approach. We do think this behaviour is linked to his early years. Fostering disabled children is not that easy at times.

Simon's greatest love is to go out for a meal. He relishes the company of adults. He doesn't have great communication skills so sometimes struggles in his peer group.

After Simon had been with us for a couple of years we received a phone call from stepmum informing us that Simon's birth mum had come to visit and asking if Simon could meet her. This request came out of the blue. We didn't know what to do for the best. It was time for a Planning Meeting to decide the best course of action. We had a chat to Simon who had not seen his real Mum for some considerable time. It was decided that any initial contact with Mum had to be held on his patch. He decided he would call his real Mum by her first name. A tea time visit would then be held at our house supervised by ourselves. The visit went well but Simon did not see his mum again!

'I'M LOVING ANGELS INSTEAD'

"See, I am sending an angel ahead of you to guard you along the way." Exodus23:20

Shortly after Ruby had arrived, my own belief system began to change. I had, over the years dipped into various belief systems and religions. I had been a born again Christian, a Baptist etc. As I matured, the church mattered less to me and, yet, I was seeking and was curious about spiritual difference.

Eventually I felt a nudge towards being attuned as a Reiki Healer. Life has enhanced this as, time and time again, when we found ourselves in tricky situations, someone would arrive to help or a solution would be found. This was often involved in day to day living in the mundane patterns. We always talk about our 'parking angel.' Wherever we go there is always a space for us. I also believe that Ruby can see angels. I often witnessed her looking at a space in the room chatting away to the space and smiling. Once she had settled down, she loved going to bed and was happy to lie down and be cosy. She would then chatter away very happily. I always believed her angels were with her. She loved the energy during the healings I gave her after her massage which her Physiotherapist had shown me.

I was out at a shopping centre with one of the foster children. It was lunch time so we went to the food hall. I chose some sandwiches and ordered some cold drinks. I had my head down looking into my purse for the money to pay. I was certain I had a twenty pound note. My purse was empty I was beginning to panic slightly so my head remained down whilst I searched for my money. I was thinking to myself I will have to tell the assistant that I have no money. Then I heard a bell ringing and I looked up at the assistant who was holding a banner: *"CONGRATULATIONS LUNCH IS ON US TODAY"*. I laughed and looked skyward and whispered thank you .....The *assistant had no idea just how timely this was. I had won a free lunch!*

I believe this is the work of angels. They help us each day with anything and everything. I am so grateful to them.

It was New Years Eve. We were at home with Ruby and Simon. We had planned a quiet day with maybe a trip out for lunch depending on how we were feeling. The phone rang, it was my daughter's father-in-law (Guido) who live a few hundred miles away in London. He was ringing to ask if we could come to see the New Year in as my daughter was missing us. Guido wanted it to be a surprise for her. So we readily agreed. It would mean bringing our dog plus the children and the wheelchair. My daughter lived in a flat where the only access was up two flights of a fire escape.

So we decided to set off early tea time and arrive in time for the New Year. We were excited at doing this spur of the moment thing as we usually planned ahead. We were driving towards the motorway when the mini bus hit a bollard in the road. I had to stop on a dark road on the outskirts of the city.

We had no idea where we were or the name of the road we were on. This meant that we were unable to give the rescue service our whereabouts. I walked off to try and find a street name or some clue as to where we were. We were in quite a dilemma. So we stood outside the minibus in the pitch dark not knowing what to do next. Then a fantastic bright red sports car rolled up. The black guy inside the car was wearing so much gold round his neck and wrists. He stopped and asked if we needed help. We explained our predicament. He said: "No worries, I will be back in a short while." So off he drove and promptly disappeared. Some anxious minutes later he returned and told us the name of the road, he had had to go about half a mile to the sign at the bottom of the road to see where we were. Now we could ring and get assistance. A breakdown truck arrived twenty minutes later and towed us back home. We then set off again in some different transport. We did make it to London in time to let the New Year in with my daughter and she was thrilled to see

51

us. We managed to get Ruby and her wheelchair up the fire escape. Our pet dog, Rosie was frightened of going up steps so my son-in-law had to carry her.

I believe that the gentleman in the red car was an angel. They come in all shapes and sizes and in all guises.

'IT'S ALL OVER, NOW'
'ENDINGS 2004'

"Every raindrop that falls is accompanied by an Angel. For even a raindrop is a manifestation of being". The Prophet Mohammad

The phone was ringing.
"This is Doctor Jones" the voice said. I was eager to hear the news. Michael had recently been to the hospital for tests.
"We need to see Mr Johns urgently. Could you ask him to contact me as soon as possible."
After carefully placing the phone back, my thoughts began to race, What if this. What if that....
The results had found cancer and it would require invasive treatment.
A hospital appointment was made very quickly. He was diagnosed with Prostate Cancer. Bad news is always difficult. My first thoughts were that we were in this together, Michael needed my support. So much of our married life had been spent caring for others. Now was the time when we needed to care for ourselves and support each other. Not knowing what the outcome would be, we made the difficult decision to ask Social Services to find alternative accommodation for Ruby. This was such a difficult thing to do and absolutely heartbreaking.
Ruby had been with us for over ten years. She had grown into a lovely young lady and, of course, she had got heavier. I was also suffering myself. I was growing older and my body was beginning to feel the strain. Pushing a wheelchair over the years had begun to

52

take its toll. I was feeling tired and my bones ached quite badly. I was carrying on in spite of feeling like this because I could not bear to think of what the alternative might be for Ruby. On hearing about Michael's illness, I knew that something would have to give.

Social Services took an awful long time to find anywhere suitable. It was difficult to find accommodation that had all the facilities. Adult Services are very different to the children's service. At the time there appeared to be a lack of funding and resources although the situation has now changed for the better. We found Ruby's new social worker to be particularly unsupportive, although she was acting on behalf of her management team and had a heavy case load. I felt bad enough myself, coping with enough and feeling worried sick that I could lose my husband. We placed more and more pressure on Social Services so that Ruby eventually moved out. It really should not have been like that. Adult placements are few and far between and really good quality care was even harder to find. I cannot state how devastating this was for her. We really loved her. It was so hard. I began to understand the meaning of being between a rock and a hard place. These were dark days.

In many ways I was not ready to let go. Ruby was very much like one of my own children. She was unable to understand anything of what was going on. I was feeling exhausted with the strain.

Ruby was eventually placed in a respite unit which was far from ideal.

It was near Christmas and I went to see her one evening, I was fighting through traffic. It was snowing. I was determined to carry on with the journey to see her. It took me ages so I arrived much later than I had arranged. When I got there I spent time in her room with her. She was pleased to see me. I was trying to explain to her why ..... I felt so bad more because she could not really understand what I was saying to her. Eventually I gave up trying to be strong. I just held her and told her we would always be in her life, that she would always be a part of our family.

Ruby was in this unit for a year before a suitable home was found for her. She had begun to be increasingly upset by some of the

53

residents who came for short breaks. After visiting her new home she more or less decided on the place she wanted to be. When she was taken on visits she was reluctant to leave making it quite clear to the staff what she wanted. At home I was praying for a miracle for her that she would be placed in a lovely situation which suited her. Her new home consists of a bungalow which has wonderful staff who really care. There are three other residents and the home is small enough to be a real home for her where she can make choices and the staff listen to her and over time understand all the meanings of her behaviour. Ruby has a lovely room and garden plus a programme of activities.

The best thing is we keep in touch with Ruby. I try and spend one day at the weekend with her plus a day during the week. We take her out or sometimes she spends the day with us and enjoys a roast dinner. In lots of ways Ruby has grown up. She has formed new positive relationships. She is happy and I am absolutely thrilled that it worked out so well.

I continue to grieve for her because we let her go. The emotional pain remains. I continue to feel guilty. Sometimes she looks at me and her eyes are asking if she can come back. I can hardly bear it. I know that I would not be physically up to it. So we do what we can. I try and attend her meetings so that we are sure her needs are being met. We have learned to trust the staff.

I recently went on holiday for a few days with Ruby and a member of staff to help. It felt really nice to be together again. This was a valuable time and I am hopeful that the experience will be repeated.

As for Michael's treatment he did receive the all clear after two years. This was the end of two years of worry and stress. We are very grateful to all the specialists involved.

BOXING DAY 2008

'ANGELS FROM THE REALMS OF GLORY'
"Angels from the realms of glory.
Wing your flight o'er all the earth"
Hymn 64, Montgomery.T 'Hymns Ancient & Modern Revised.'

"Merry Christmas, Ruby. You look very smart." I gave her a big smile as Caroleanne pushed Ruby into the lounge. "Give me a kiss." Ruby reached up to her mouth with her right hand and blew me a kiss. This was a good sign and let us know she was happy to be here. Once in the lounge Ruby was greeted by a chorus of welcoming faces of members of our extended family who had assembled for our annual bash.

"Have you got some presents to open?" said my son Richard. He and his girlfriend had just arrived from their flat based in Manchester.

"Richard, Richard," Ruby replied all doe eyed as she recognised the person she had a crush on for many years.

"How are you?" said Daniel clearing a space for Ruby's wheelchair as I sorted out the drinks. I was in charge of the bar.

"Do you want a drink, Ruby?" I asked. "Does anyone else want a drink?"

"Let's have one of your quizzes later" asked Richard. "You know you're not going to win, Dad."

"You just wait and see, mate. I've been practising. We've just opened a new DVD quiz game for Christmas."

"Can't wait." said Daniel who was our current quiz champion.

I charged everyone's glasses handing Ruby a glass of lemonade.

"Pop, pop," she giggled beaming as she recognised all the people sat in the lounge. Ruby's smile could melt an iceberg.

"Dinner won't be long." yelled Caroleanne through two sets of doors. "Why don't you give Ruby the 'Christmas TV Times' she'll enjoy that." Ruby was happy to flick through a magazine as she likes the feel of the paper between her fingers and enjoys flicking over the pages again and again. She then progressed on to some new jigsaws we had brought her for Christmas

"Can I do anything to help, love?" I could smell the turkey and roast pork from the corner of the lounge.

"You could wheel Ruby in and then ask everyone to sit down," said Carole.

The traditional lunch started off with the loud bang of crackers being pulled. Simon loved helping to pull everyone else's as he liked to save the toys inside.

As Simon helped to pull Sara's cracker she said: "Daniel and I are planning to take you to a theme park later in the year. Would you like that?"

"That will be great." Simon replied. He loved his last visit to Alton Towers accompanied by Daniel and his fiancé who were nearer his age.

Ruby had no problems finishing off all her dinner. She loves lots of meat and gravy as long as it's not too hot.

"Would you like some more, Ruby?" asked Caroleanne.

"Caroleanne, Caroleanne, more," said Ruby. This was a definite yes.

After lunch everyone went into the lounge to exchange presents. Ruby had arrived carrying a bag full of gifts.

"Shall I help, you?" Caroleanne asked as she took out the presents one by one. "Simon you can help and hand these to people."

"This is lovely, Ruby. Thank you."

"Thanks Ruby. I like the colour a lot."

"What have you got, Caroleanne?"

"It's some nice perfume."

"Do you want some help with opening yours, Simon?"

The room gradually filled up with sheets of coloured paper as everyone opened their gifts. Simon piled all his presents onto a chair making the perfect photo opportunity. He then offered to help clear up all the mess. This was the cue to start the quiz. We finished in fits of laughter as we have a tradition of making sure that Daniel's team wins. Later in the game, Simon spotted Ruby's care staff park outside the house in their minibus. It was sadly time for her to return back to her hostel.

"We're going into town for a nightcap, Richard, do you and Rachael want to join us?" asked, Daniel. "We've arranged to meet up with Gav."

"Shall we go, Rachael?" pleaded Richard.

"Why not?"

Within the space of half an hour Caroleanne and I were left on our own. This meant we had all the clearing up to do. It was a family tradition you know!

The room was strangely quiet as Simon sat in the corner gazing at all his presents.

I started to reflect on the last twelve years thinking of all of our achievements. "We've had a lovely day, Caroleanne. Do you remember last Christmas when we all went out to that place on the Chevin? What a great time we had"

"Have you enjoyed yourself, Simon?" asked Caroleanne.

"Yes," muttered Simon who was looking tired.

"Let's take all your presents up to your room. We can play with some of them tomorrow." I escorted Simon up to his room. "Ruby will be back in a couple of days. So you will see her then."

"It's been a lovely Christmas, Michael. Let's watch some TV and then go to bed. I'm looking forward to seeing Ruby next week." said Caroleanne as we both slumped into the comfort of our settee.

"Merry Christmas, Michael." said Caroleanne raising a glass of wine.

"Merry Christmas, love," I replied, "let's have a toast to the New Year. Cheers!"

USEFUL INFORMATION

FOSTERING

Fostering is looking after someone else's child in your own home as part of your family. The child has a care plan that details the care they need. A key aspect of a Professional Foster Carer is to work with the foster child's birth family. You are also part of a team that is caring for the child. All our children had an allocated Social Worker whose role was to visit the child on a regular basis.

Some children are unable to live with their birth families, therefore, their case is referred to a Court of Law and a Care Order is imposed by the terms of 'Children's Act 1989'. In some cases a child can become 'accommodated' under voluntary arrangements with the child's parents.

You will also be involved with working with: Health professionals, hospital consultants, speech and language therapists, Child Psychiatrist, Special Educational Needs Co-ordinator to name but a few.

'*Fostercare*' *childrens.service@hants.gov.uk*)

Caroleanne and I wanted to do something that really made a difference to children's lives. Our reward was to feel that we helped to create a brighter future for disabled children who came to stay.

We began to understand the world from a child's point of view. We quickly learnt that a child who comes into care has a limited understanding of what is happening to them. Some children will act out their anger and frustration that is inside them.

Our job was to find a way for a child to express their feelings in a positive way. We had to find time to listen to the child and stick with them through difficult patches in their lives. (Bond H (2004))

We discussed strategies with our Link Worker and also attended relevant training courses on behaviour management.

FAMILY PLACEMENT

When we had decided to become foster parents we approached a local Family Placement Service. This scheme pay an allowance and offer preparation, training and ongoing support. The scheme recruits people who are willing to offer their home to care for children with disabilities. We were appointed a Link Worker who was extremely supportive and was able to sort out most problems.

In the initial interviews our Link Worker explained that there were several options open to us. The short term placement scheme seemed to be our best option whilst we saw how we got on. Ruby arrived about a year later we were able to apply for a transfer onto their Long Term Scheme.

EQUAL OPPORTUNITIES

I attended courses on the subject of Equal Opportunities and it was always a topic that came along at interviews as there was always a question aimed at testing your knowledge of this subject. The subject came more alive when Ruby came to stay. We had to find ways that would help her become acquainted with the West Indian part of her heritage. Her hair required specialist care and every year we attended the local carnival. During this event Ruby was able to sample the sights and sounds of various cultures which may be connected in some way with her own. Ruby used to enjoy 'Jerk Chicken' served from the many stalls. Our link worker at Family Placement introduced us to a volunteer who was a black worker who offered to befriend Ruby. She would come and visit Ruby on many occasions and this became an example of 'good practice' which became a hall mark for the work that 'Family Placement' did.

OUR APPROACH:
LIFE STORY BOOKS

Life story book work is aimed at helping children in foster care come to terms with their relationships of the past. It is regarded as a form of healing and reconciliation. Life story book work gives a child a structured and understandable way of talking about situations that happened to them. In our case we completed the exercise for both Ruby and Simon, by obtaining birth certificates and old photographs and placing them in chronological order. (It is vital to keep copies of all information that has been collected as some children will destroy it) We also kept photographic records of holidays plus other memorable occasions.

The completed life story book follows the child throughout their journey. For more information: Ryan T and Walker R, "Life Story Work" A 'Practical guide to helping children understand their past' (2007) BAAF Adoption and Fostering.

We thought we might share a few ideas that worked for us. The plans work better when discussed with a team.

'STAR CHARTS'

This is one method of behaviour modification that we used to help us deal with some challenging behaviour.

We purchased an exercise book with graph pages and a packet of different coloured star stickers. The next step is to identify the behaviour you are trying to change. It is advisable to choose ONE at a time.

In the back of the book complete a list of rewards which could include: chocolate, time on the computer, extensions to bed time, trip to McDonald's etc. The rewards are decided in discussion with the child and previous carer. Every child will have different preferences. The emphasis here is on praise rather than punishment. Then decide on a time frame before a star is allocated. In some cases the time frame could be as short as ten minutes before awarding a star. It can easily be extended at any time.

(Some children can get themselves into a "punishment cycle" and can't find a way out of it. They are set up to fail unless they are helped.)

Three blue stars followed by a gold star equal a reward. Depending on the child's understanding, after two gold stars a larger reward is given. This system helped us in our initial days as foster carers and we witnessed many improvements in children's behaviour. Some became totally involved in achieving a gold star in order to receive the reward. In order to help a child who had enuresis we placed a large sheet of card above his bed. On the morning the child was dry he was allocated a blue star. After two blue stars he was allocated a gold star, this triggered a reward. After three gold stars we all went to the 'Pizza Hut' and brought him a milkshake. It worked!

BEHAVIOUR PLAN

First allocate an amount of spending money the child receives each week.

In our case the child received seven pounds per week, therefore, he was allocated one pound per day.

Each evening spend some time with the child to discuss the day and talk about any difficulties and problems they have experienced.

A bedtime story is selected and, in our case, it was important to maintain some consistency and read to the child every night. This part of the plan is very important and must NEVER be cancelled.

Give lots of praise during the day in order to encourage. We found that it was important to tell a child he was being good and NOT wait for him to do something naughty. Some will in order to gain attention.

If there are any serious discipline issues then ten pence is deducted from the daily allowance which he should receive every night at bed time.

"If you use that swear word again I will deduct ten pence from your daily allowance". Give a warning beforehand.

At bedtime explain that they can start again the following day from scratch. "Tomorrow is a new day and we will start again."

PLEASE NOTE all fines deducted are saved in a money box and used to purchase bigger treats to use as a reward when the behaviour improves or is consistently good over a period of time.

You could do a list of behaviours you are trying to discourage but focus on one at once.

Keep a log to measure the behaviour. DO NOT get into a situation where the child receives no money at all.

Invite the child to do jobs around the house to earn extra money.

Make a list of rewards before commencement of plan. If the chosen behaviour improves over one week then implement a reward: MacDonald's, CD, comic etc. This plan should be reviewed at regular intervals and shouldn't really be carried on indefinitely. Try it for a month.

FORMAL BEHAVIOUR PLAN

'Therapeutic Crisis Intervention' by Martha J Holden and Beth Laddin from: 'The Family Life Development Centre, College of Human Ecology Cornell University Ithaca, NY (1998)

This behaviour plan was utilized by to Leeds City Council from America and we were introduced to this method by attending a training course. The course had been adjusted to suit a fostering environment.

HOLIDAY INFORMATION

This is some information on the holiday companies we used. There are plenty of people willing to help. We are not making any recommendations as some of the options can be more expensive than planning holidays yourself. We have had some wonderful holidays with all of these.

- 'Enable Holidays' lists over 30 properties in holiday destinations that are accessible. Contact 0871 222 4939 www.enableholidays.com
- 'The Scout Holiday Homes Trust.' list of self catering caravans and chalets all based in UK. Contact: 020 8433 7100 www.scouts.org.uk/holiday homes.
- 'CanbeDone' offers a wide range of accommodation all over the world as well as information on coach tours which always use adapted vehicles. It provides details of accommodation in London and other cities in the UK.
  Contact: 020 8909 1854 www.canbedone.co.uk.
- 'Eurocamp' provides fully equipped tents with a fitted kitchen based on sites throughout Europe, Greece, Denmark and the USA. They all have a free 'Kids Club' on site. Contact: 0844 499 1499 www.eurocamp.co.uk.
- 'Keycamp' provides fully equipped tents across Europe and the USA. Also provides Chalets and Mountain lodges but the tents are the most accessible in our experience. A good tip is to check on the access to the swimming pool on each site. Free 'Kids Club' on site.
  Contact: 0844 844 1000 www.keycamp.co.uk.

Bibliography

Useful publications referred to during our fostering years.
Argent H. *'What is a disability?' 'A guide for children.'*
Explains in simple language and pictures what life is like for a disabled child. (2004) BAAF
Bond H. *'Fostering a child' 'A guide for people interested in fostering'* (2004) BAAF
This book tells you what you need to know about fostering. It includes a list of all the independent fostering providers.

Brading J.and Curtis J. *'Disability Discrimination.' 'A Practical Guide to the New Law.* (2000) Kogan Page Limited.

Cairns K. *'Attachment, trauma and resilience' 'Therapeutic caring for children'* (2009)BAAF
Kate Cairns is a Social Worker who has fostered 12 children. The book describes scenarios of how her family responded to children who displayed powerful feelings and difficult behaviour.

Elliot M' and Kilpatrick J. *'How To Stop Bullying: A Kidscape Training Guide'* (1994) Kidscape, London.
Information and exercises for people interested in helping to tackle bulling.

Honos-Webb, L. *'The Gift of ADHD' 'How to Transform Your Child's Problems into Strengths'* (2005) New Harbinger Publications Ltd.
This book is intended for parents of children who are six to twelve years old and have been diagnosed with attention-deficit/hyperactivity disorder. Written in language we could understand.

Klein N. *'Healing Images for Children' 'Teaching Relaxation and Guided Imagery to Children Facing Cancer and Other Serious illnesses'* (2000) Inner Coaching, Wisconsin.

Marsden R. *'The Family Business' 'The story of a family's adoption of a boy with cerebral palsy'* (2008)
Robert Marsden is a Social Worker who describes his own experience of adopting a child who is a wheelchair user. He describes incidents that were very similar to our own.

Palmer I. *'What to Expect When You're Adopting'* (2009) Vermilion, London

Ryan T. and Walker R. *'Life Story Work' 'A practical guide to helping children understand their past.* (2008)BAAF See 'Useful Information'
British Association for Adoption & Fostering (BAAF)
Skyline House, 200 Union Street, London SE1 0LX
www.baaf.org.uk
An organisation that has an extensive list of other publications